MW00876419

THE 15 ANTI INFLAMMATORY HERBAL REMEDIES TO KNOW BEFORE 2024

Eliyah Mashiach

Disclaimer

The information provided in this book by Eliyah Mashiach is for general informational purposes.

UNDER NO CIRCUMSTANCES SHALL WE BE LIABLE TO YOU FOR ANY LOSS OR DAMAGE OF ANY KIND INCURRED AS A RESULT OF YOUR USE OF THE SITE,
OR DEPENDENCE ON ANY INFORMATION CONTAINED ON THIS SITE, OR USE OF ANY INFORMATION CONTAINED ON THIS SITE OR BOOK. USING THE INFORMATION PROVIDED IS SOLELY AT YOUR OWN RISK.

Table Of Contents

Introduction

Greetings everyone!!! I am Eliyah Mashiach a Natural Herbalist. In this book, I will be sharing with you all 39 anti-inflammatory herbal remedies that you can make at home, which will benefit you, the entire family as well as your neighbors. I truly hope that you will find each remedy beneficial to the area/s that you need.

What Is Inflammation

Inflammation is a natural process by which the body remove harmful stimuli and heal itself. Inflammation is a very important part of protecting the body from harmful irritants, stimuli, pathogens and even damaged cells. In simple terms, inflammation is a natural function of our body's defense system/mechanism. It is important to note that inflammation is designed by our Heavenly Father to let us be aware that something is wrong within our bodies. As a result, once the process of inflammation has started certain signs can be clearly seen, observed and noted. These signs include:

- Pain in or around the affected area
- Swelling
- Redness/discoloration
- Loss of function/numbness
- Warmth/heat

With these clear signs above, we generally should have knowledge and understanding of when we are inflamed or when inflammation is present. I urge us to be more in tuned with our bodies and to be more aware of when something is not right or does not feel normal within our bodies. It is also important to pay keen attention to the area of the body where inflammation is present. Though inflammation is a natural part of the body's natural defense system to initiate healing, we must know that chronic inflammation can lead to sickness, excessive discomfort and even death. Once the body's defense system starts to work, we should be aware, so we can give assistance to the body and the immune system in order to speed up healing and recovery.

For example, an object fell on your toe. The moment you start feeling the pain you should become aware and seek to render assistance to the body's natural defense system, in order to help speed up healing and recovery. This means, instead of leaving the body's defense system solely to work on the toe, you would soak your affected toe/foot in warm sea salt water for a few minutes, then you would dry properly and massage your toe with rosemary oil. The above example is the prescribed way to hinder and prevent an inflammation from becoming a chronic inflammation. Bear in mind, if we are not aware of what is happening in and with our bodies, the possibilities and risk of chronic inflammation will be higher/greater.

Chronic Inflammation

Chronic inflammation is an inflammation that lasts for long periods of time. This kind of inflammation can last for several months, years, or even a lifetime. As stated earlier, it is important to monitor the body's normal defense mechanism (inflammation) and assist in helping the body to have a speedy recovery. Having this type of practice will help to hinder or prevent the development of chronic inflammation.

Chronic inflammation leads to chronic illnesses/diseases and chronic illnesses/diseases can lead to a life of misery, frustration, torment, discomfort, exorbitant money spending, embarrassment, lack of self-confidence, fear, doubt, mistrust, disrespect, depression, anxiety and sadly, even death. With all that is said above, we give Yahweh thanks for giving us all the herbs necessary to help prevent and heal chronic inflammation.

For centuries, herbal remedies have been used to prevent and remove chronic inflammation while enabling the body to properly heal itself. It is important to note that, herbal remedies are very effective in getting rid of the root of the chronic inflammation. In addition to this, when you can identify where in the body the inflammation is, it becomes much easier to treat the inflammation, with the right herbs. For example, if you start to wheeze and start experiencing shortness of breath, you should now realize that there is an inflammation in the bronchial tubes and the respiratory system. Once you have identified where the inflammation is, you now must use the right herbs specifically designed to remove the inflammation from that part of the body. Removing chronic inflammation can be very simple, but it takes consistency and a strong pursuit to heal yourself. It simply means that changes to lifestyle habits, practices and diet may have to be done.

Many people would want to be miraculously healed, which mean they would rather to do nothing at all to aid in their recovery but rather to be awaken the next day to find out that their chronic inflammation, illnesses/diseases are all gone. It must be noted that the above is possible and will be happening, however, with the information in this book and other truthful information out there, lays the platform and the solid foundation for us to work in treating our own sicknesses and the sicknesses of others.

In this book we will cover 39 anti-inflammatory herbal remedies that will help you, your family and your neighbors. There are more information that will be given in other books that I will publish soon, but for now, let us look carefully through these 39 anti-inflammatory herbal remedies. Pleasant reading!

Brain/Neuro - Inflammation

Brain inflammation naturally occurs when the body's natural defense system attends to an infection or injury in the brain. Depending on how chronic the infection or injury is, chronic inflammation can occur. When chronic inflammation exists in the brain, several health problems, illnesses, conditions or diseases can occur as a result. These include but not limited to:

- Alzheimer's disease
- Stroke
- Depression
- Parkinson's disease
- Anxiety
- Epilepsy
- Fibromyalgia
- Headaches/migraines
- Autoimmune disease etc.

At this point, we should have a better understanding of what brain inflammation is and what can occur when chronic inflammation exists in the brain.

In the following pages we will look at some natural remedies to help hinder, prevent or remove brain inflammation.

Remedy 1

Boil in 4 cups of water for 10 mins, 2 teaspoons of sage and 2 teaspoons of rosemary.

Strain and drink 2-3 cups a day.

Remedy 2

Boil in 4 cups of water for 10 mins, 1 tablespoon turmeric and 1 tablespoon of ginger.

Add a pinch of black pepper.

Strain and drink 2-3 cups a day.

Remedy 3

Steep in 1 cup of hot water for 10 mins,

½ teaspoon ginkgo biloba powder.

Drink 2 cups a day.

Remedy 4

Boil in 4 cups of water for 10 mins, 1 sprig of rosemary and 2 teaspoons of ashwagandha.

Strain and drink 2-3 cups a day.

Remedy 5

Blend in 2 ½ cups of water, ¼ cup of sea moss

2 teaspoons of sage and juice from 1 lime.

Strain, add honey (optional) and drink throughout the day.

Remedy 6

Steep in 4 cups of hot water for 10 mins, 1 sprig of rosemary and 2 tablespoons of ginger.

Strain and drink 2-3 cups a day.

Respiratory Inflammation

As the heading suggest, this is an inflammation that affects the lungs, bronchial tubes, airways and eventually our ability to breathe properly. Respiratory inflammation often cause excessive mucus to build up, tightening of the chest, coughing, wheezing, and difficulty breathing. In addition to this the sinuses and nasal passages can become inflamed. As a result, a person experiencing respiratory inflammation, can experience stuffiness and congestion.

Respiratory inflammation that is left untreated or unattended, can lead to chronic respiratory inflammation. Chronic respiratory inflammation include but not limited to:

- Asthma
- Bronchitis
- COPD
- Chronic Rhinitis
- Chronic Sinusitis etc.

In the following pages we will look at some natural remedies to help hinder, prevent or remove chronic respiratory inflammation.

Remedy 1

Boil in 4 cups of water for 10 mins, 2 teaspoons of licorice root and 2 teaspoons of mullein.

Strain and drink 2-3 cups a day.

Remedy 2

Boil in 4 cups of water for 10 mins, 4-6 oregano leaves and 2 tablespoons of ginger.

Strain and drink 2-3 cups a day.

Remedy 3

Boil in 4 cups of water for 10 mins, 1 sprig of thyme and 1 sprig of peppermint.

Strain and drink 2-3 cups a day.

Remedy 4

Steep in 4 cups of hot water for 10 mins, 3 teaspoons of eucalyptus leaves and 1 tablespoon of grated ginger.

Strain and drink 2-3 cups a day.

Remedy 5

Boil in 4-6 cups of water for 10 mins, 1 purple onion, 4 chopped garlic cloves, 1 tablespoon chopped ginger and 1 teaspoon cayenne pepper.

Strain and drink 2-3 cups a day.

Remedy 6

Steep in 4 cups of hot water for 10 mins, 1 sprig of thyme,

1 tablespoon of grated ginger and 2 teaspoons of mullein.

Strain and drink 2-3 cups a day.

Joint Inflammation

Joint inflammation can occur as a result of wear and tear, injury, infection, or autoimmune disorders. When joints are inflamed they become swollen, stiff, difficult to move,, and painful. Chronic joint inflammation can lead to the following:

- Rheumatoid arthritis
- Psoriatic arthritis
- Osteoarthritis
- Gout etc.

In the following pages we will look at some natural remedies to help hinder, prevent, or remove chronic joint inflammation.

Remedy 1

Boil in 3 cups of water for 10 mins, 2 teaspoons of nettle leaves, and 1 teaspoon of devil's claw.

Strain and drink 2-3 cups a day.

Remedy 2

Boil in 4 cups of water 1 tablespoon cat's claw, 2 teaspoons of Boswellia and 1 teaspoon grated ginger.

Strain and drink 2-3 cups a day.

Remedy 3

Boil in 4-6 cups of water for 10 mins, 2 tablespoons of willow bark, 1 teaspoon turmeric powder, 2 tablespoons grated ginger and a pinch of black pepper.

Strain and drink 2-3 cups a day.

Remedy 4

Boil in 4 cups of water for 10 mins, 2 teaspoons of devil's claw and 2 teaspoons of turmeric. Add a pinch of black pepper.

Strain and drink 2-3 cups a day.

Remedy 5

Boil in 4-6 cups of water for 10 mins, 2 tablespoons willow bark and 1 tablespoon of Boswellia.

Strain and drink 2-3 cups a day.

Remedy 6

Steep in 2 cups hot water for 10 mins, 1 teaspoon turmeric powder and 1 teaspoon of grated ginger. Add a pinch of black pepper. Strain and drink 2 cups a day.

Skin Inflammation

Skin inflammation occurs as a result of allergic reactions, infections, auto immune disorders, injury etc.

When the skin is inflamed it becomes swollen, irritated, red, itchy, dry or flaky. Chronic skin inflammation include but not limited to:

- Psoriasis
- Rosacea
- Seborrheic dermatitis
- Lichen planus
- Chronic acne etc.

In the following pages we will look at some natural remedies to help hinder, prevent or remove chronic skin inflammation.

Remedy 1

Boil in 4-6 cups of water for 10 mins, 3 teaspoons calendula and 3 teaspoons licorice root.

Strain and drink 2-3 cups a day.

Remedy 2

Boil in 4-6 cups of water for 10 mins, 3 teaspoons of chamomile, 3 teaspoons of calendula and 1 tablespoon of chopped ginger.

Strain and drink 2-3 cups a day.

Remedy 3

3 teaspoons neem leaves, 2 teaspoons ginger, 4 teaspoons calendula and 3 teaspoons turmeric. Combine all ingredients and use 1 heaping teaspoon to 1 cup of hot water. Let sit for 5 minutes, strain and drink once per day.

Remedy 4

Boil in 4-6 cups of water for 10 mins, 2 teaspoons gotu kola, 2 teaspoons sage and 2 teaspoons chamomile.

Strain and drink 2-3 cups a day.

Remedy 5

Boil in 4-6 cups of water for 10 mins, 3 teaspoons of lemon balm, 2 teaspoons of dandelion root and 2 teaspoons of burdock root.

Strain and drink 2-3 cups a day.

Remedy 6

Steep in 3 cups of hot water for 10 mins, 2 teaspoons of yarrow flower and ½ teaspoon of cayenne pepper.

Strain and drink 1-3 cups a day.

Note briefly: Neem oil, calendula oil, comfrey ointment, garlic oil, tea tree oil and aloe vera, can be used for skin care.

Circulatory Inflammation

Circulatory inflammation occurs within the blood vessels of the body. This inflammation affect the capillaries, veins and arteries. Chronic circulatory inflammation can lead to:

- Heart failure
- Damage to the lungs
- Numbness in limbs
- Cramping
- Fatigue
- Weakness
- Cardiovascular disease
- Stroke
- Decreased blood flow
- Plaque in the arteries
- Clots in the blood
- Damaged kidneys etc.

In the following pages we will look at some natural remedies to help hinder, prevent, or remove chronic circulatory inflammation.

Remedy 1

Steep in 2 cups of hot water for 10 mins, 1 teaspoon of gingko biloba and ¼ teaspoon cayenne pepper.

Strain and drink 2 cups a day.

Remedy 2

Boil in 4 cups of water for 10 mins, 2 teaspoons skullcap leaves and 2 teaspoons of hawthorn.

Strain and drink 2-3 cups a day.

Remedy 3

Boil in 4 cups of water for 10 mins, 1 tablespoon of dried horse chestnuts seeds and 2 teaspoons of St. John's wort.

Strain and drink 2-3 cups a day.

Remedy 4

Boil in 6 cups of water for 10 mins, 3 teaspoons licorice root and 3 teaspoons of chamomile.

Strain and drink 1-3 cups a day.

Remedy 5

Boil in 6 cups of water for 10 mins, 1 sprig of basil, 2 tablespoons of grated ginger and 1 tablespoon of turmeric root.

Strain and drink 2-3 cups a day.

Remedy 6

Boil in 4-6 cups of water for 10 mins, 2 tablespoons of green tea leaves and 2 tablespoons of hibiscus flowers.

Strain and drink 2-3 cups a day.

Remedy 7

Boil in 4 cups of water for 10 mins, 1 tablespoon cat's claw, 2 teaspoons of Boswellia and 1 teaspoon grated ginger.

Strain and drink 2-3 cups a day.

Remedy 8

Boil in 4 cups of water for 10 mins, 2 tablespoons of rosemary and 2 tablespoons of gotu kola leaves.

Strain and drink 2-3 cups a day.

Muscle Inflammation

Muscle inflammation occurs when there is inflammation in the muscles. This cause muscle swelling, fatigue, numbness, soreness, weakness and muscle pain. Muscle inflammation can occur as a result of but not limited to:

- Infection
- Flu
- Wear and tear
- Injury
- Overuse
- Strain
- Sprain
- Auto immune disorders etc.

In the following pages we will look at some natural remedies to help hinder, prevent or remove chronic muscle inflammation.

Remedy 1

Boil in 4 cups of water for 10 mins, 1 tablespoon of grated ginger and 2 teaspoons of dried milk thistle seeds.

Strain and drink 2-3 cups a day.

Remedy 2

Boil in 4 cups of water for 10 mins, 2 tablespoons slippery elm powder and 4-5 oregano leaves.

Strain and drink 2-3 cups a day.

Remedy 3

Boil in 6 cups of water for 10 mins, 1 ½ tablespoons of devil's claw powder and 1 ½ tablespoons wild yam root.

Strain and drink 2-3 cups a day.

Remedy 4

Steep in 4 cups of hot water for 10 mins, 3 teaspoons of nettle and 1 sprig of thyme.

Strain and   drink 2-3 cups a day.

Remedy 5

Boil in 4-6 cups of water for 10 mins, 3 teaspoons horsetail herb, 3 teaspoons calendula and 1 tablespoon grated ginger.

Strain and drink 2-3 cups a day.

Remedy 6

Boil in 4-6 cups of water for 10 mins, 2 teaspoons of grated turmeric root, 2 teaspoons of grated ginger and 1 teaspoon of licorice root.

Strain and drink 2-3 cups a day.

Remedy 7

Blend ¼ cup aloe vera with 1 cup coconut water. Drink 1 cup in the morning consistently for 7 days.

Note Briefly: Natural oils and ointments made from comfrey, thyme, oregano, lavender, cayenne pepper, rosemary, eucalyptus, chamomile, neem and ginger, can be used to massage inflamed muscles.

Conclusion

The 39 Anti- Inflammatory Herbal Remedies To Know Before 2024 as you have read, is carefully formulated for my readers to have a clear and concise understanding and insight into these powerful, simple, and natural anti-inflammatory herbal remedies that can be of great benefit to you, your family and to your neighbors. These remedies are so simple, and these ingredients can be found in your kitchen cabinet, your garden, your nearby herbal store, or local markets.

Many people would want to be miraculously healed, which mean they would rather to do nothing at all to aid in their recovery but rather to be awaken the next day to find out that their chronic inflammation, illnesses/diseases are all gone. It must be noted that the above is possible and will be happening, however, with the information in this book and other truthful information out there, lays the platform and the solid foundation for us to work in treating our own sicknesses and the sicknesses of others. After all your health is still your wealth.

We have more books on the way and we ask for your continued support as we bring helpful and informative information and knowledge to you in this time of **climatic changes**. May our heavenly father Yahweh Elohiym and our savior Yahshua Ha Mashiach guide you on this journey to long life. Shalohm

Notes

Made in the USA
Las Vegas, NV
22 December 2023

83444864R00017